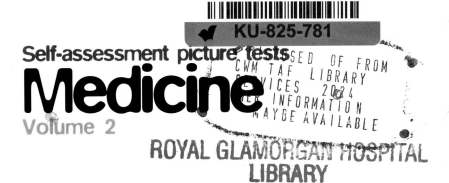

Self-assessment picture tests
Medicine
Volume 2

Pierre-Marc Bouloux
BSc MD FRCP

Reader in Endocrinology
Department of Endocrinology
Royal Free Hospital
London

E11898

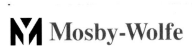

London • Baltimore • Barcelona • Bogotá • Boston
Buenos Aires • Carlsbad, CA • Chicago • Madrid
Mexico City • Milan • Naples, FL • New York
Philadelphia • St. Louis • Seoul • Singapore
Sydney • Taipei • Tokyo • Toronto • Wiesbaden

Mosby-Wolfe

Publisher:	**Richard Furn**
Development Editor:	**Jennifer Prast**
Project Manager:	**Linda Horrell, Jane Tozer**
Production:	**Gudrun Hughes**
Index:	**Angela Cottingham**
Layout:	**Lindy van den Berghe**
Cover Design:	**Greg Smith**

ISBN 0 7234 2465 9   Set ISBN 0 7234 2468 3

For full details of all Times Mirror International Publishers Limited titles, please write to Times Mirror International Publishers Limited, Lynton House, 7–12 Tavistock Square, London WC1H 9LB, England.

A CIP catalogue record for this book is available from the British Library.

Preface

Much of clinical practice consists of pattern recognition, and the ability to detect swiftly and interpret physical signs correctly is at the heart of the diagnostic process (and indeed a prequisite for passing clinical examinations!). In these four volumes, I have compiled 800 examples of common and not so common clinical problems covering wide areas of medicine. The format is simple, unambiguous and unpretentious: a photographic plate with a short question, or questions, relating to the physical sign or underlying diagnosis. The aim is to challenge the reader's diagnostic skills. I have annotated the answer in many cases to give the reader some background information about the condition illustrated. These volumes should be seen as an adjunct to existing illustrated textbooks of clinical medicine such as Forbes/Jackson *Color Atlas and Text of Clinical Medicine,* 2nd edition.

Acknowledgements

I would like to acknowledge the wonderful assistance given to me by the Department of Medical Illustrations at the Royal Free Hospital School of Medicine, and the excellent support of Miss Patsy Coskeran in assembling the material.

To Jane, Dominic, Matthew, Natalie and my late brother Alain

1 ▶

(a) What lesion is shown?

(b) List three associations.

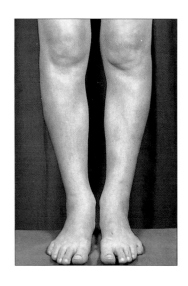

2 ▶

This patient was under treatment for tuberculosis and developed a photosensitive eruption. What diagnosis is suggested?

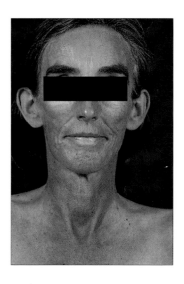

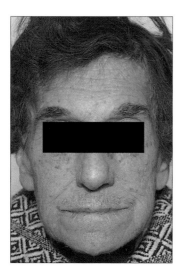

◄ 3
This lady complained of dysphagia. What is the diagnosis?

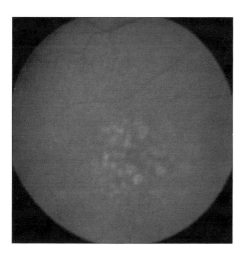

◄ 4
This is the fundal appearance of a patient with gradually declining visual acuity. What is the diagnosis?

5 ▶
What is the cause of this
appearance?

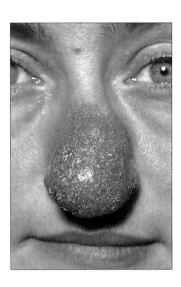

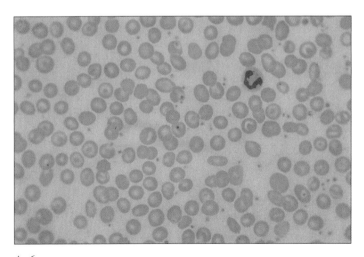

▲ 6
What abnormalities are seen on this blood film?

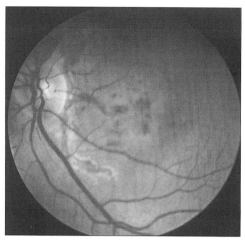

▲ 7
(a) What physical sign is shown?
(b) List two associations.

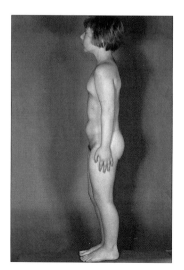

◄ 8
This young girl was investigated for primary amenorrhoea and short stature. What is the likely cause?

9 ▶

This man complained of gradual deformity of his nose. Suggest two possible causes.

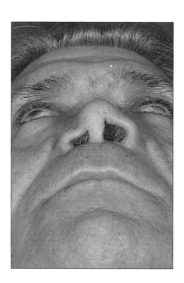

10 ▶

What is the diagnosis?

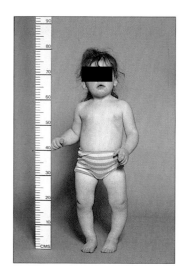

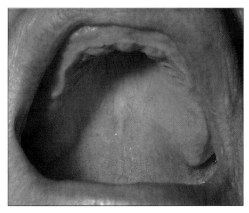

▲ 11

This man had a pneumothorax. This appearance was found on routine examination.

(a) What physical sign is shown?

(b) What is the underlying diagnosis?

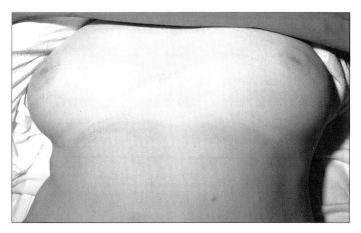

▲ 12

These are the breasts of a patient with an XY karyotype, in whom there was a striking absence of pubic hair. What diagnosis is suggested?

13 ▶

Despite aspiration of this lesion, it kept recurring. What is the most likely diagnosis?

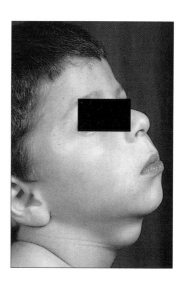

14 ▶

What physical sign is shown?

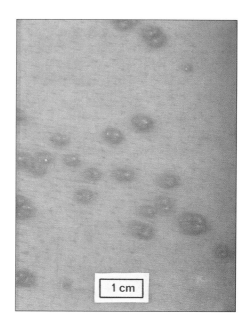

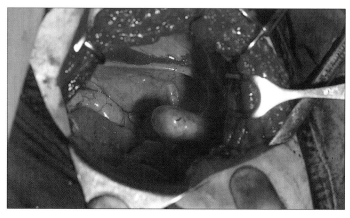

▲ 15

These are the laparotomy findings of the patient in **12**. What abnormality is shown?

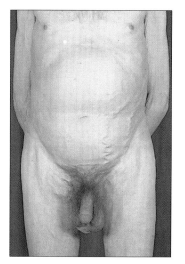

◀ **16**

This patient had a myeloproliferative disorder. What may have caused the appearance of this abdominal wall?

17 ▶

This is the appearance of the skin of a patient who was totally asymptomatic, but developed gradually spreading and coalescing lesions from her toes up to her buttocks. Urinalysis was negative, there was no fever, and the blood film was normal. What is the most likely cause of this purpuric rash?

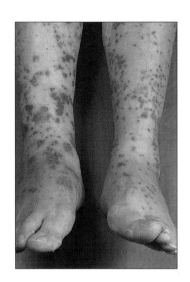

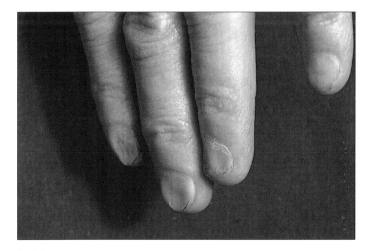

▲ **18**

(a) What physical sign is shown?

(b) With what abnormality is it associated?

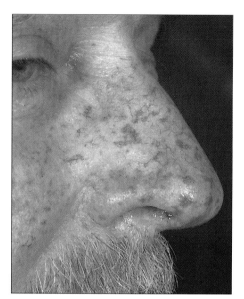

This is the nose of a patient under investigation for chronic iron deficiency. What is the diagnosis?

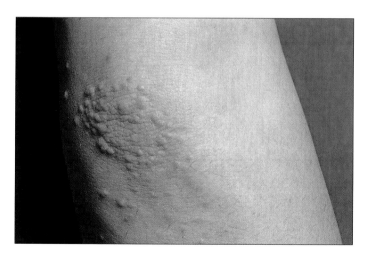

▲ 20
(a) What is the most likely cause of these appearances?
(b) What investigation is indicated?

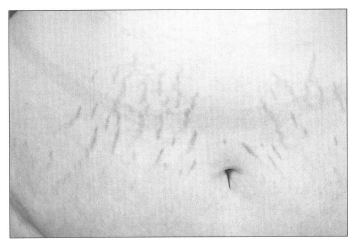

▲ 21
(a) What physical sign is shown?
(b) List two associations.

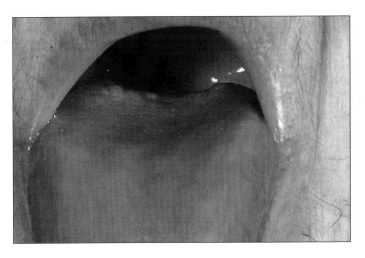

▲ 22
(a) What physical sign is shown?
(b) What investigation is indicated?

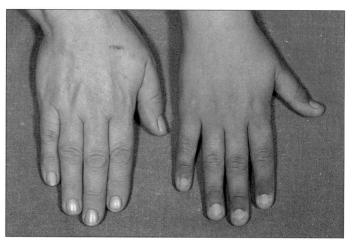

▲ 23
The hand on the right is from a young man receiving regular blood transfusions. What physical sign is shown?

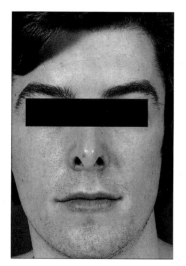

◀ 24
This patient has always had clinically obvious cyanosis, but was totally asymptomatic. What is the most likely diagnosis?

25 ▶
This young man was receiving regular transfusions for a chronic anaemia. What is the most likely diagnosis?

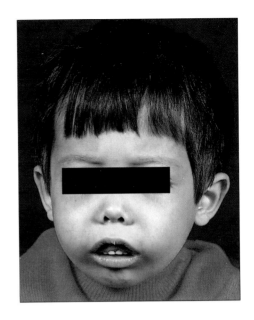

26 ▶
This is the appearance of a patient with acute lymphoblastic leukaemia who had been treated by bone marrow transplantation. What is the likely cause of this appearance?

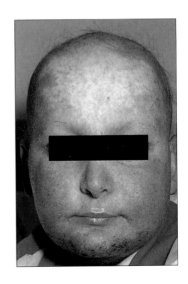

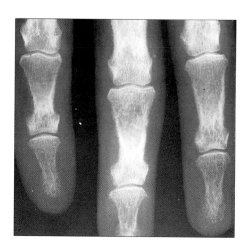

◄ 27
This is a radiograph of a patient under investigation for polyuria and polydipsia.
(a) What abnormality is shown?
(b) What biochemical abnormality is likely to be present?

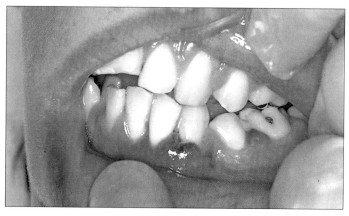

▲ 28
(a) What abnormality is shown?
(b) List three possible causes?

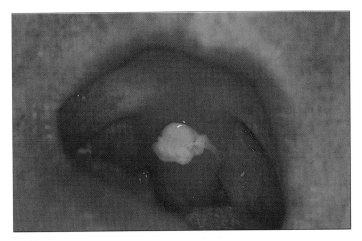

▲ 29
This is the mouth of a patient under treatment for acute myeloid leukaemia.
(a) What physical sign is shown?
(b) What is the treatment?

30 ▶
This methylene diphosphonate technetium scan was undertaken in a patient with hip pain. What is the likely diagnosis?

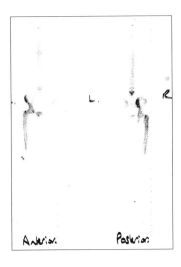

Anterior.   Posterior.

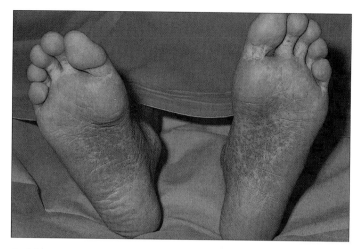

▲ 31

These are the feet of the patient shown in **26**. What is the likely diagnosis?

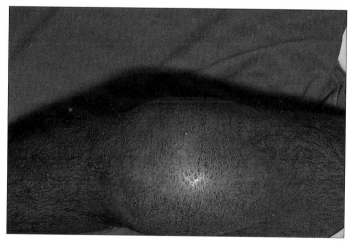

▲ 32

Following a relatively minor injury this patient developed a sudden extremely painful swelling of his knee. There had been several such episodes in the past. What is the likely diagnosis?

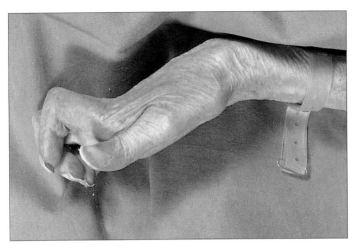

▲ 33

This patient suffered major trauma to his arms several years before. What diagnosis is shown?

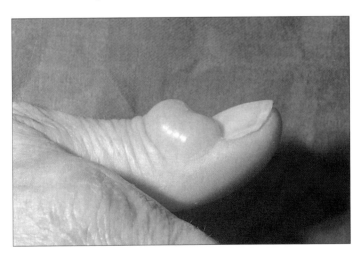

▲ 34

What is the likely cause of this appearance?

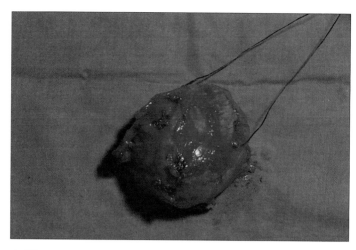

▲ 35
This is the adrenal resection specimen from a patient with episodic severe hypertension. What is this most likely to be?

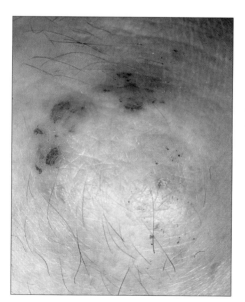

◄ 36
This is the elbow of a patient with intense itching, weight loss, and diarrhoea. What is the most likely diagnosis?

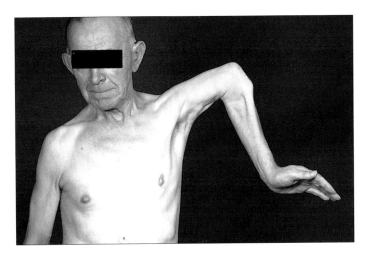

▲ 37

What abnormality is shown?

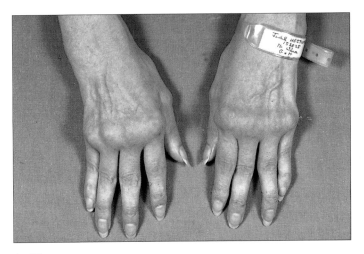

▲ 38

(a) What physical signs are shown?

(b) What is the diagnosis?

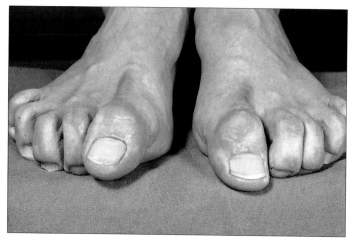

▲ 39
(a) What physical sign is shown?
(b) List three associations?

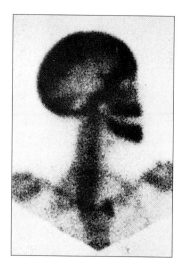

◄ 40
What abnormality is shown on this technetium bone scan?

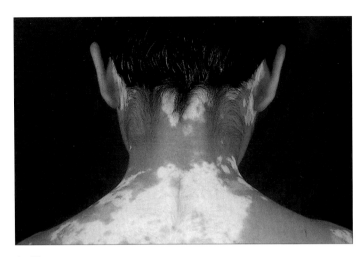

▲ 41
(a) What physical sign is shown?
(b) List two associations.

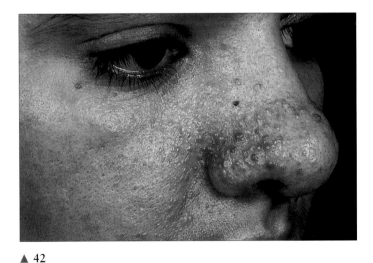

▲ 42
(a) What physical sign is shown?
(b) With what neurological abnormality is it associated?

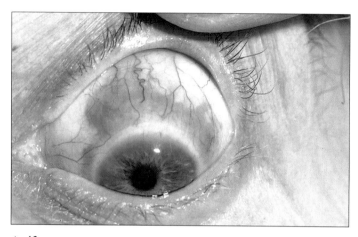

▲ 43
(a) What lesion is shown?
(b) What are the associations?

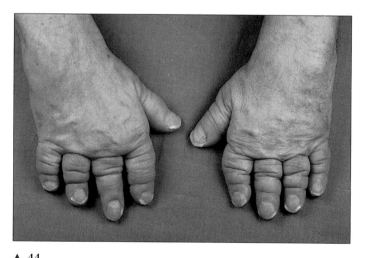

▲ 44
(a) What physical sign is shown?
(b) What is the likely underlying diagnosis?

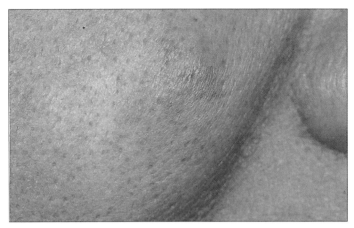

▲ 45
This chronic lesion was present in a patient under investigation for fever, hypercalcaemia, and nocturia. A number of lesions were present around the eyelids. What is the most likely diagnosis?

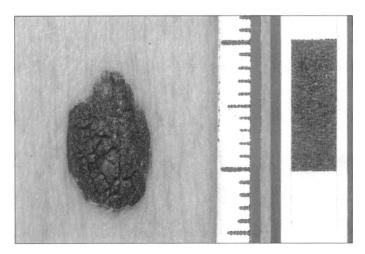

▲ 46
This lesion had been present for a number of years. What is the most likely diagnosis?

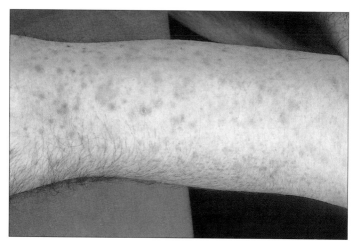

▲ 47
These lesions were itchy and had been present for many years.
What is the diagnosis?

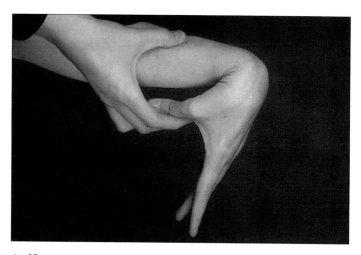

▲ 48
(a) What physical sign is shown?
(b) List two associations.

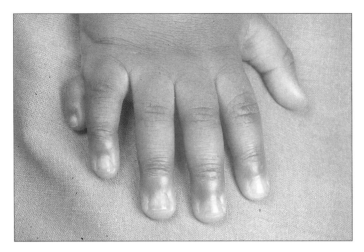

▲ 49
(a) What physical sign is shown?
(b) With what may it be associated?

50 ▶
(a) What physical
    sign is shown?
(b) The patient had
    blue sclerae.
    What is the most
    likely underlying
    diagnosis?

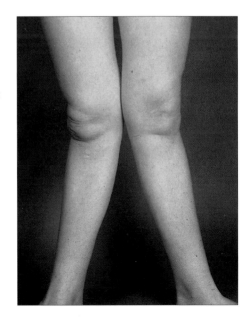

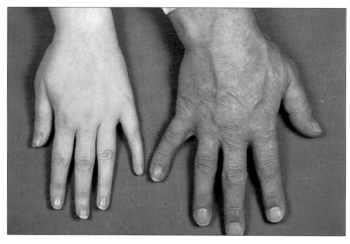

▲ 51
The larger discoloured hand (a control hand is shown for comparison) is that of a patient with diabetes mellitus and abnormal liver function tests. What is the likely diagnosis?

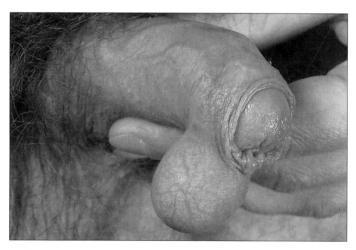

▲ 52
This lesion had been present from birth. What is it?

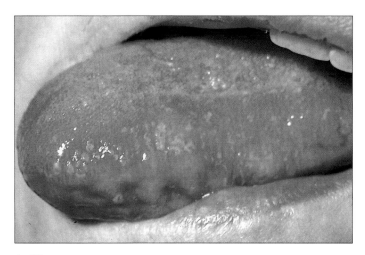

▲ 53
(a) What lesion is shown?
(b) List one important association.

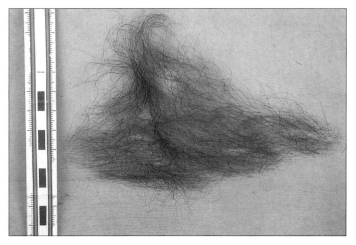

▲ 54
This lesion had been present since birth. What is it?

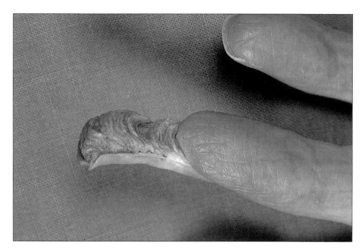

▲ 55
What physical sign is shown?

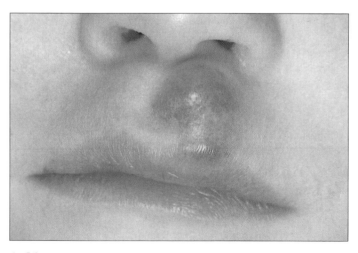

▲ 56
This lesion had been present since birth. What is it?

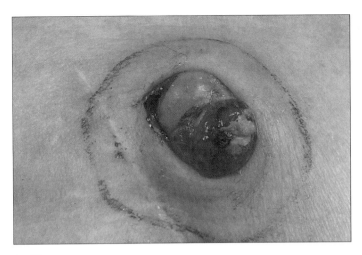

▲ 57
This chronic lesion had been present within the umbilicus for over five years. What is it?

58 ▶
This patient complained of sudden monocular loss of vision. What is the likely cause?

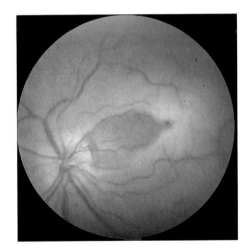

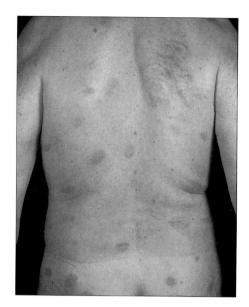

◀ 59
These lesions were
widespread,
particularly over the
back and the flexor
surface of the arm,
where they were
itchy and irritating.
What is the
diagnosis?

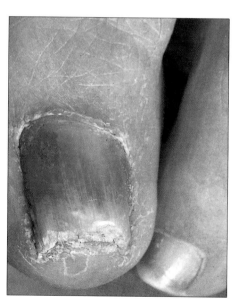

◀ 60
(a) What lesion is
   shown?
(b) Suggest one
   possible
   treatment.

61 ▶

These are the arms of a young man under treatment for a pancytopenia. What is the diagnosis?

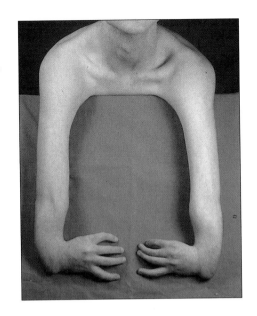

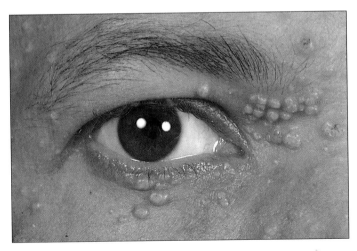

▲ **62**

What is the diagnosis?

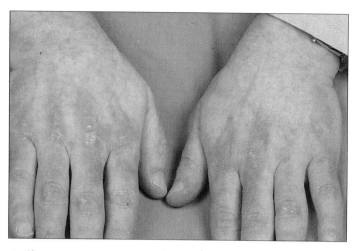

▲ 63
What lesion is demonstrated on the dorsum of these hands?

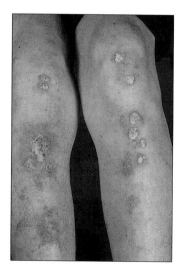

◀ 64
What is the diagnosis?

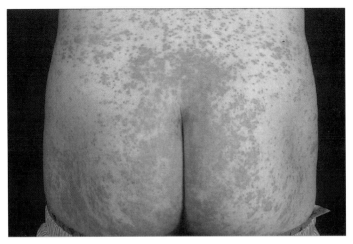

▲ 65
This eruption appeared in a patient who complained of abdominal pain and had traces of haematuria on urinalysis. What is the likely diagnosis?

66 ▶
What lesions are shown on the front of this man's chest?

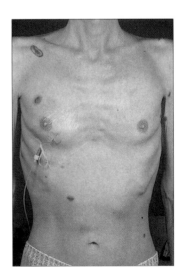

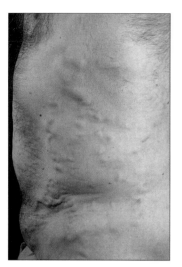

◀ 67
This is the abdominal wall appearance in a patient who had presented with ascites and tender hepatomegaly and spenomegaly eight months previously. Jaundice was present initially. What is the likely diagnosis?

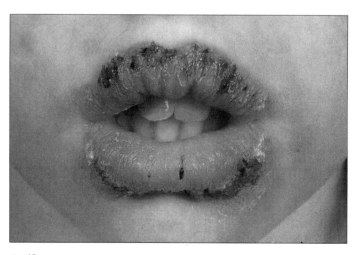

▲ 68
What lesion is shown?

69 ►

This patient complained of a sudden altitudinal visual field loss.
(a) What is the diagnosis?
(b) What is the likely underlying cause?

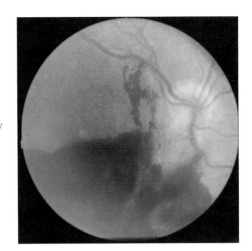

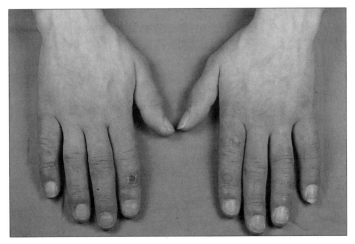

▲ **70**

This man complained of painful hands, particularly in the cold weather. What lesions are shown?

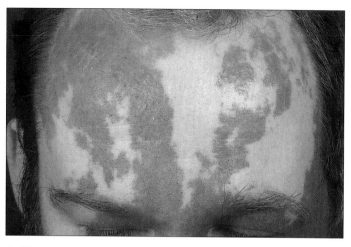

▲ 71
(a) What physical sign is shown?
(b) What treatment may be given?

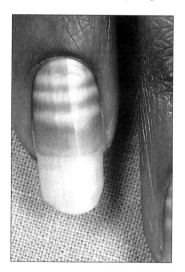

◄ 72
What physical sign is shown?

73 ▶

What physical sign is shown?

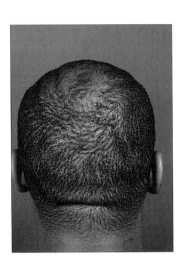

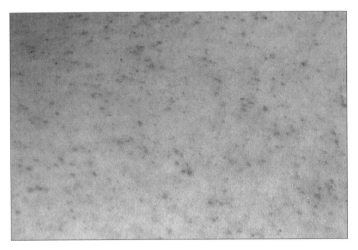

▲ 74

These lesions appeared over a period of days, and did not blanch. The patient also complained of nose bleeds. What physical sign is shown?

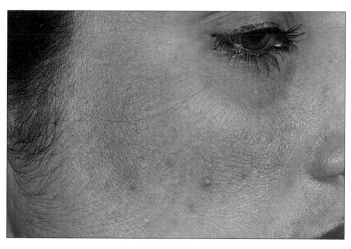

▲ 75
This patient was taking an oral contraceptive pill. What physical sign is shown?

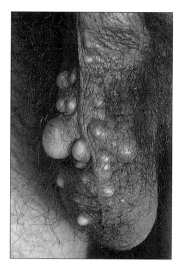

◀ 76
What is the likely cause of the appearance of this man's scrotum?

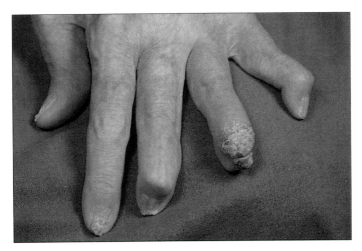

▲ 77
What unifying diagnosis would account for the appearances of this hand?

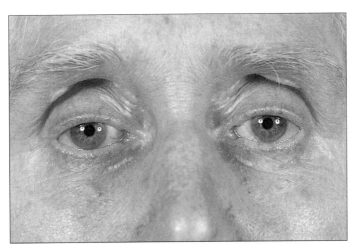

▲ 78
List two physical signs seen in this patient.

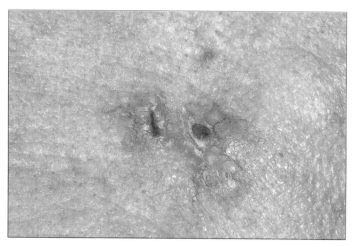

▲ 79

This lesion had been present for over one year, and bled periodically. What is the diagnosis?

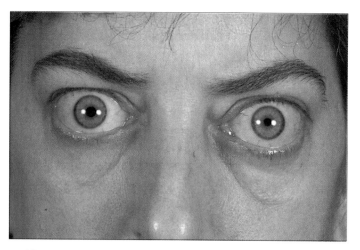

▲ 80

(a) What physical sign is shown?
(b) With what disease is it associated?

81 ▶

This lesion had been present for six months, and bled periodically. It was slowly getting bigger. What is the diagnosis?

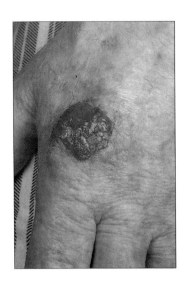

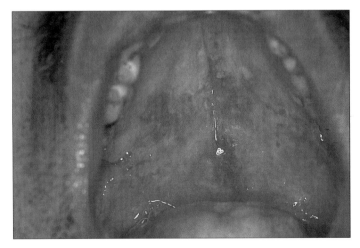

▲ 82

These oral lesions were present in a man who had a pruritic eruption with extensive denudation of the skin. What is the diagnosis?

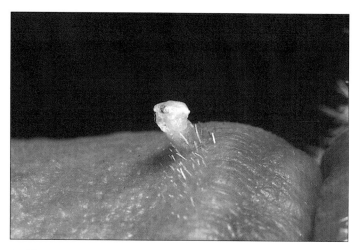

▲ 83
What lesion is shown?

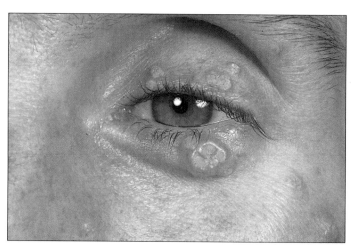

▲ 84
What lesion is shown?

85 ▶

This man complained of a midline lesion above his laryngeal prominence that moved on swallowing. It had been there virtually all his life. What is the most likely diagnosis?

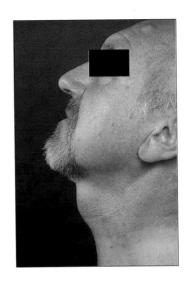

86 ▶

What physical sign is shown?

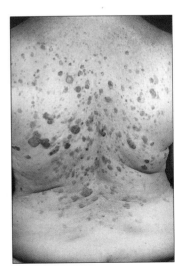

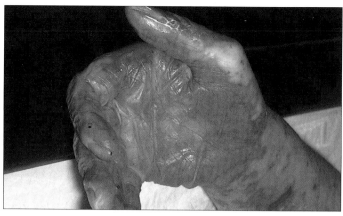

▲ 87
This skin disorder occurred about eight days after a patient had started a non-steroidal anti-inflammatory agent. What is the likely diagnosis?

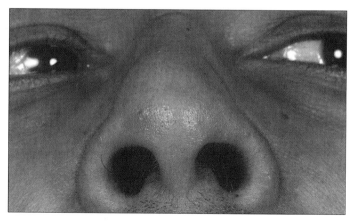

▲ 88
This patient had hypercalcaemia. What is the most likely underlying cause based on the demonstrated physical sign?

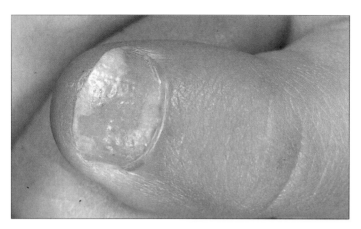

▲ 89
What is the diagnosis?

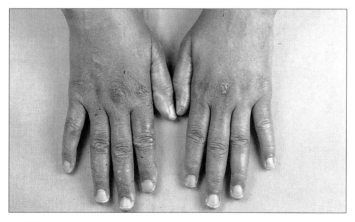

▲ 90
This patient first presented with a pericarditis and had fluffy cotton wool spots on ophthalmoscopy. Subsequently, a rash appeared on the dorsa of the hands. What is the most likely diagnosis?

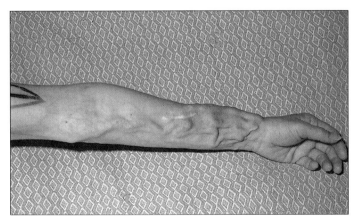

▲ 91
What is the most likely cause of this appearance?

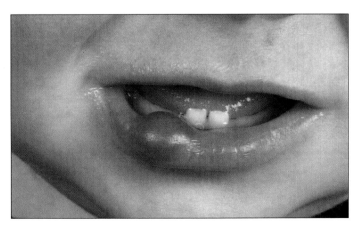

▲ 92
What is the diagnosis of this long-standing painless lesion?

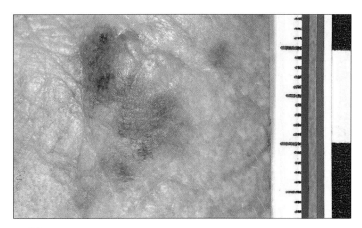

▲ 93
What physical sign is shown?

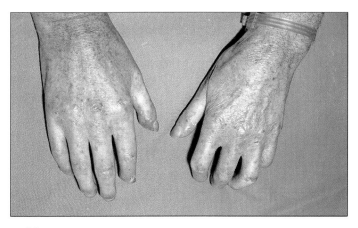

▲ 94
This patient was complaining of dysphagia. What diagnosis is suggested by the appearance of his hands?

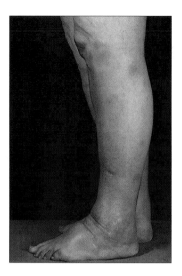

The lesions shown on the shins were tender and had developed suddenly. What is the most likely diagnosis?

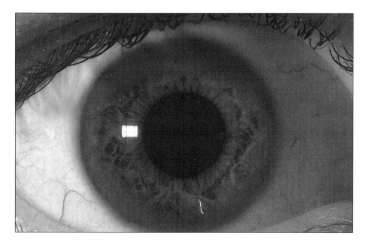

▲ 96
(a) What physical sign is shown?
(b) What is the underlying diagnosis?

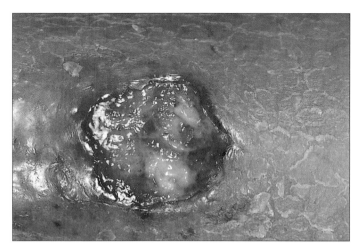

▲ 97
This lesion first started off as a tender papular lesion, which gradually broke down into a shallow ulcer over a period of two weeks. The patient was complaining of bloody diarrhoea. What is the diagnosis?

98 ▶
The lesions shown were well-demarcated plaques of firm tissue and were found only on the skin. What is the diagnosis?

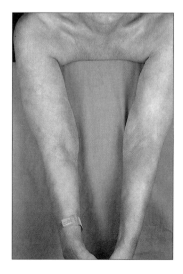

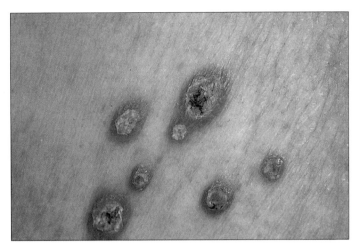

▲ 99
This crop of lesions appeared in a dermatome distribution. What is the diagnosis?

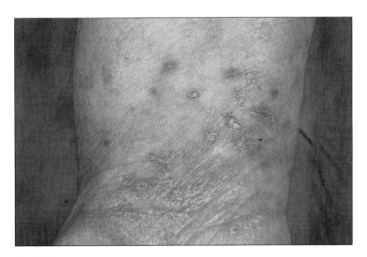

▲ 100
What is the likely cause of these intensely itchy papular lesions?

101 ▶

List two special causes of this
appearance.

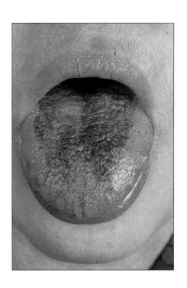

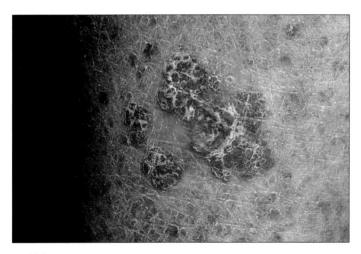

▲ **102**

This lesion was spreading superficially and gradually getting larger.
What is the likely diagnosis?

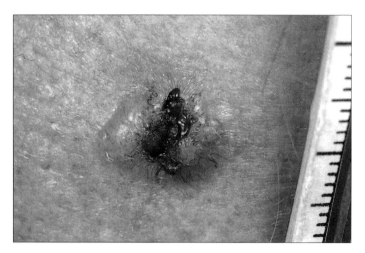

▲ 103
What lesion is this?

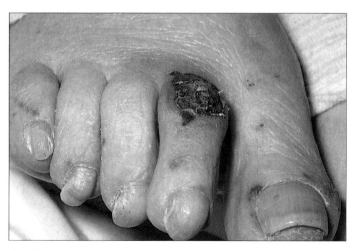

▲ 104
What is the most likely origin of these lesions?

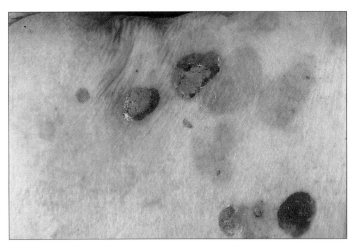

▲ 105
These lesions were previously bullous. What is the most likely diagnosis?

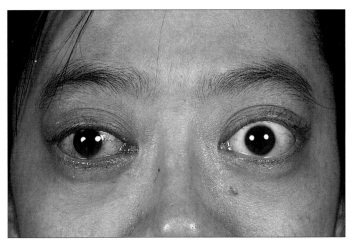

▲ 106
What diagnosis is suggested by this appearance?

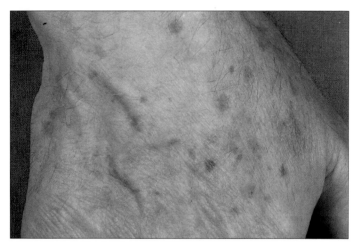

▲ 107

What is the nature of the lesions shown on the dorsa of the hands of this elderly person?

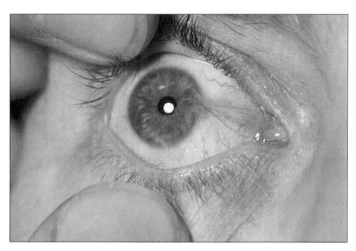

▲ 108

What physical sign is shown?

109 ▶

What is the most likely cause of this chronic lesion?

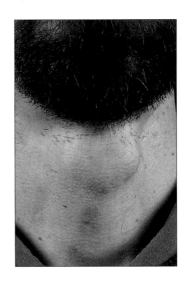

110 ▶

This girl was ten years old when this photograph was taken. She presented at birth with ambiguous genitalia and clitoromegaly, and developed hirsutes from the age of five. Breast development is rudimentary and she has not yet menstruated.

(a) What diagnosis is suggested?
(b) List two confirmatory investigations.

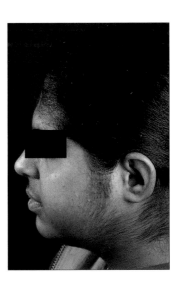

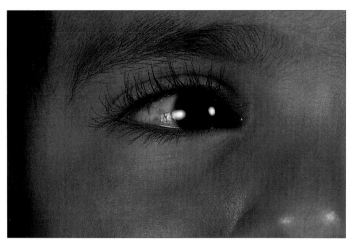

▲ 111
What physical sign is shown?

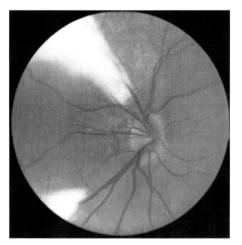

◀ 112
What is the cause of this appearance, which was longstanding and asymptomatic?

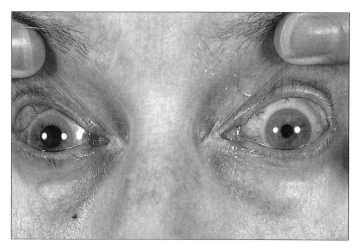

▲ 113
This patient had rheumatoid arthritis. What ocular lesions are shown?

114 ▶
This man was being treated for severe arthritis.
(a) What physical sign is shown?
(b) What is the likely underlying diagnosis?

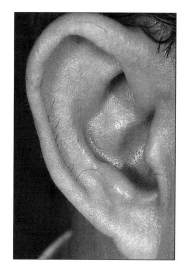

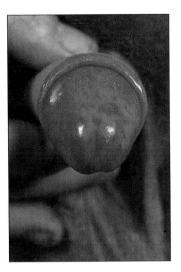

This man complained of polyuria and polydipsia. What is the likely cause of this penile appearance?

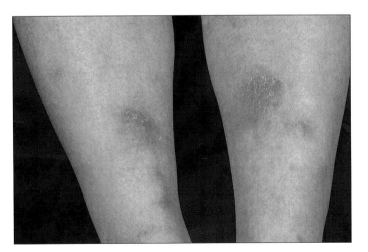

▲ 116
These lesions started off as indurated nodules on the back of the legs and gradually spread. They were painless. What is the likely diagnosis?

117 ▶
What cutaneous lesion is
demonstrated?

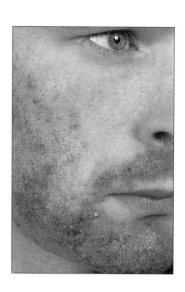

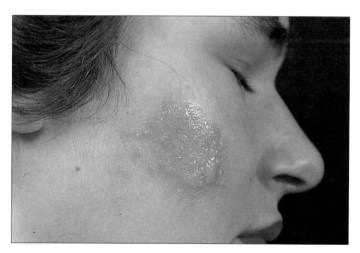

▲ 118
What is the diagnosis?

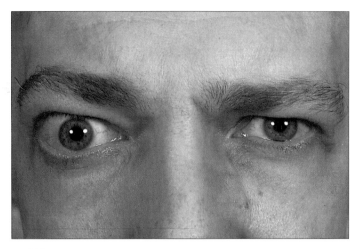

▲ 119
What is the likely cause of this appearance?

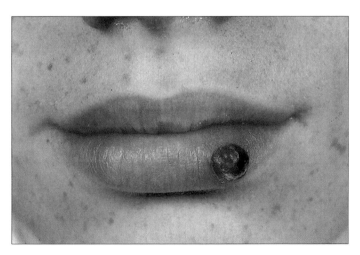

▲ 120
This lesion had been present for eight months. It bled occasionally.
What is the most likely diagnosis?

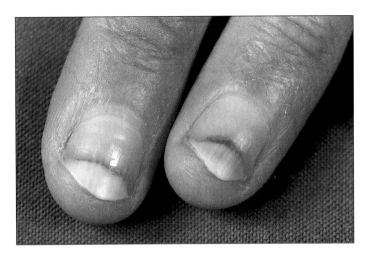

▲ 121

(a) What physical sign is shown.

(b) List two associations.

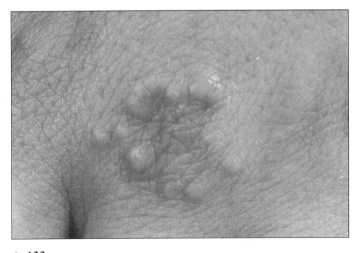

▲ 122

(a) What is the most likely cause of this appearance?

(b) How may it be treated?

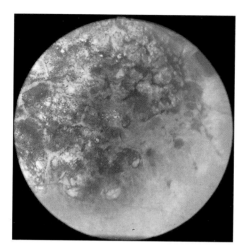

◄ 123
What is the likely
cause of this fundal
appearance?

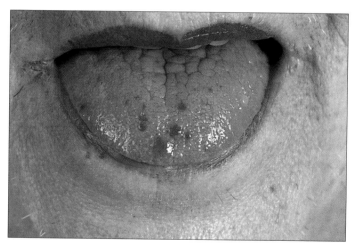

▲ 124
What underlying diagnosis would be expected from this
appearance?

125 ▶
(a) What lesions are
shown?
(b) What is the most
likely underlying
diagnosis?

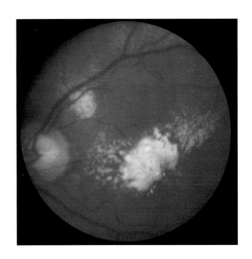

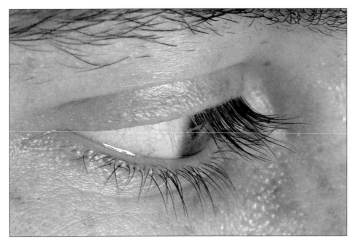

▲ 126
What physical sign is shown?

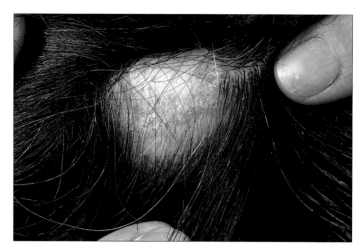

▲ 127
A cicatricial lesion can be seen on the floor of this abnormality.
What is the most likely cause?

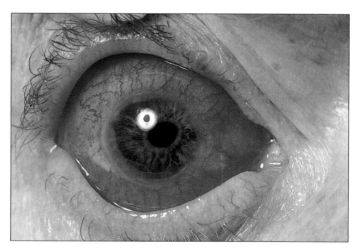

▲ 128
What is the diagnosis?

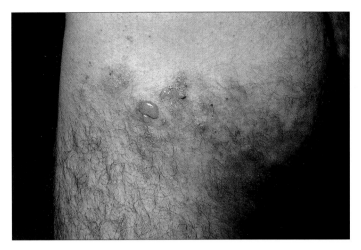

▲ 129
These intensely pruritic lesions were present on the elbow as well as on the buttocks of this individual. There was a history of diarrhoea. What is the most likely diagnosis?

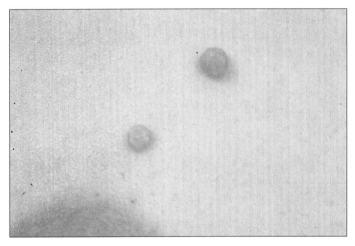

▲ 130
What is the diagnosis?

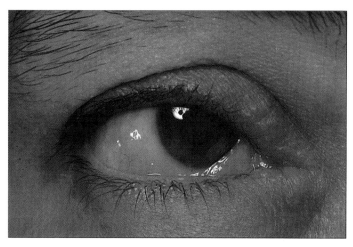

▲ 131
These lesions had been present over a long period of time and were asymptomatic. What is the most likely diagnosis?

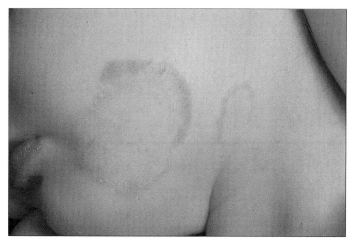

▲ 132
What is the diagnosis?

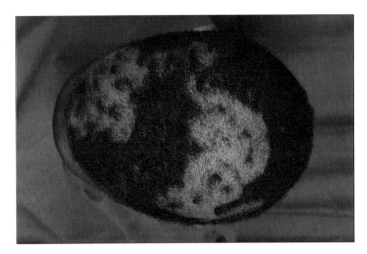

▲ 133
What is the most likely cause of this appearance?

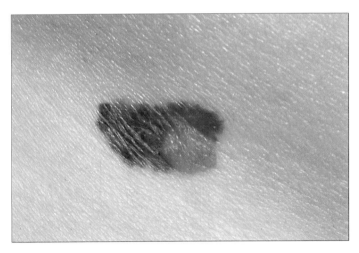

▲ 134
What is the most likely cause of this lesion?

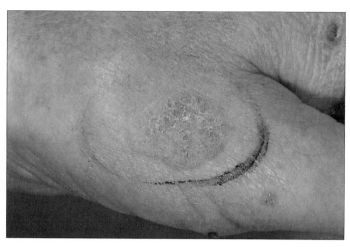

▲ 135
This lesion had been present for a twelve-month period and was
slowly increasing in size. What is the most likely diagnosis?

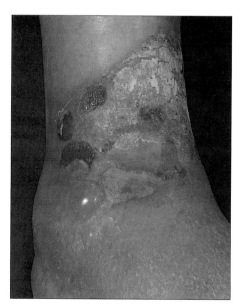

◄ 136
Other similar
lesions were present
on the thigh of this
patient. The patient
also had mucosal
involvement,
particularly of the
palate of the mouth.
What is the most
likely diagnosis?

137 ▶
(a) What lesion is
shown?
(b) What is the
underlying
biochemical
abnormality?

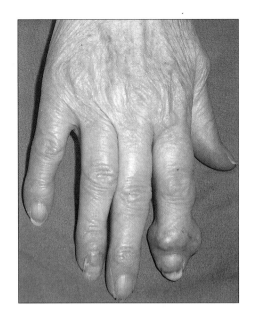

138 ▶
(a) What physical
sign is shown?
(b) List two
associations.

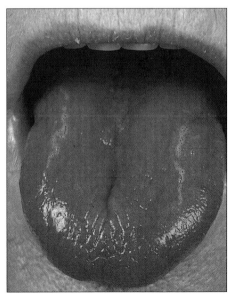

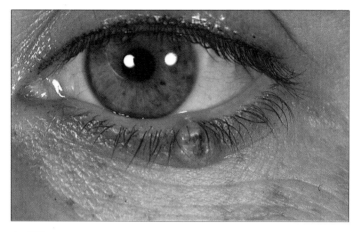

▲ 139
This lesion had been present for two years and was slowly getting bigger. There were no other similar lesions elsewhere. What is the most likely diagnosis?

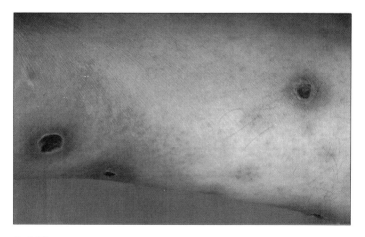

▲ 140
This patient presented with necrotic lesions over her lower limbs. She had haematuria and a high ESR. What is the most likely diagnosis?

141 ▶
What lesions are shown on fundoscopy?

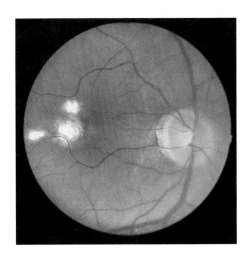

142 ▶
(a) What is the diagnosis?
(b) What visual field defect may be associated with the chronic form of this lesion?

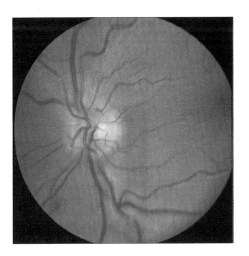

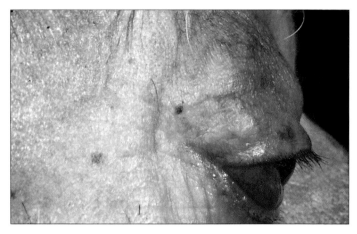

▲ 143
This patient presented with multiple purpuric lesions over the face, and particularly around the orbits, and also had heavy proteinuria, and a motor neuropathy. Suggest the likely cause of this appearance.

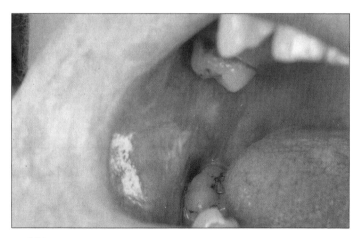

▲ 144
This oral lesion was associated with a highly pruritic eruption elsewhere in the body. What is the diagnosis?

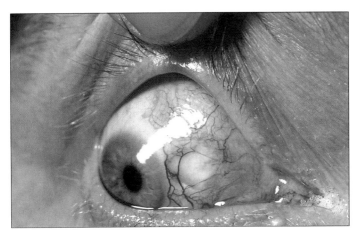

▲ 145
What is the likely cause of this appearance?

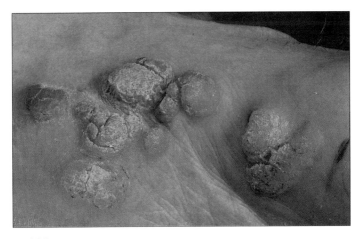

▲ 146
(a) What is the diagnosis?
(b) List two possible therapies.

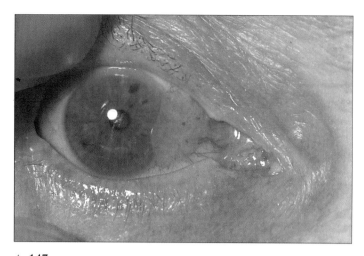

▲ 147
(a) What lesion is shown?
(b) What treatment is indicated?

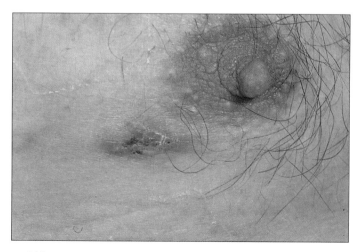

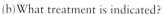

▲ 148
This lesion was present over a nine-month period in a man who had come back from a safari holiday. What is the most likely diagnosis?

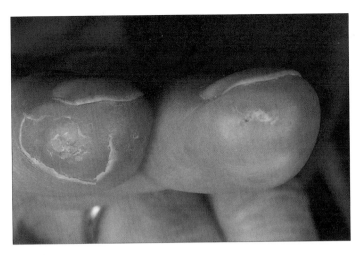

▲ 149
(a) What physical sign is shown?
(b) List two associations.

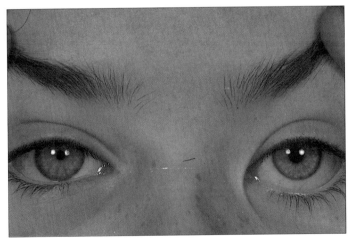

▲ 150
The patient was asymptomatic. What physical sign is shown?

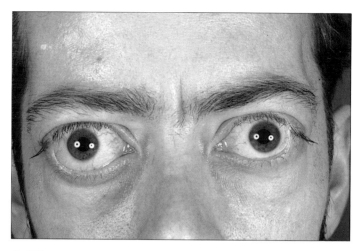

▲ 151
(a) List three physical signs in this patient.
(b) What is the likely underlying diagnosis?

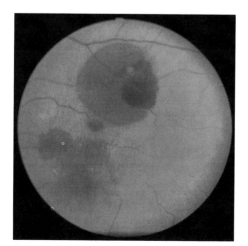

◄ 152
This patient complained of acute loss of central vision. Proteinuria was present. What is the underlying diagnosis?

153 ▶

This is the fundal appearance of an asymptomatic patient. What is the likely underlying diagnosis?

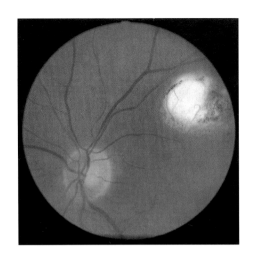

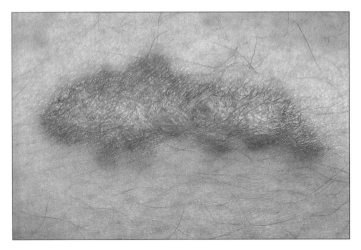

▲ 154

This lesion was found on the skin of a 32-year-old man complaining of weight loss and general debility. What is the likely diagnosis?

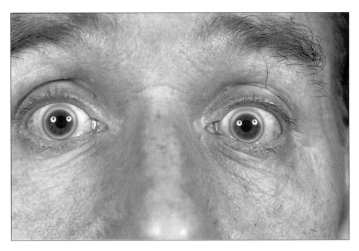

▲ 155
(a) What physical sign is shown?
(b) With what biochemical abnormality is it associated?

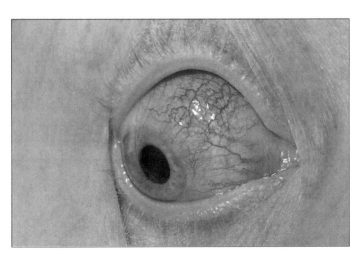

▲ 156
This patient had rheumatoid arthritis. What lesion is shown?

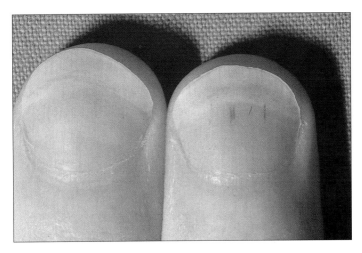

▲ 157

(a) What physical sign is shown?

(b) What is the most likely underlying diagnosis?

158 ►

(a) What is the diagnosis?

(b) What is the likely cause of the scar?

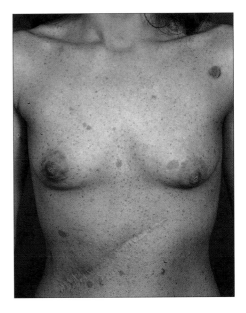

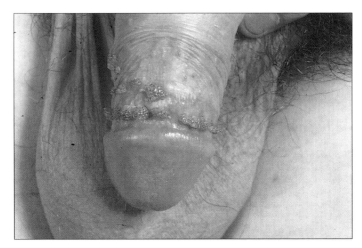

▲ 159

What is the diagnosis?

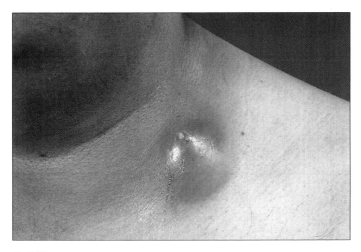

▲ 160

This lesion had been present for some months and was gradually getting larger. Eventually it discharged some pus. The patient complained of vague fevers and general ill health. What is the most likely diagnosis?

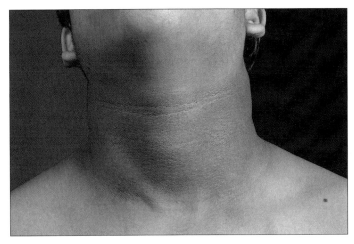

▲ 161
(a) What physical sign is shown?
(b) List three associations.

162 ▶
This is the ocular appearance of a child who developed progressive renal failure, with nephrogenic diabetes insipidus. What is the likely diagnosis?

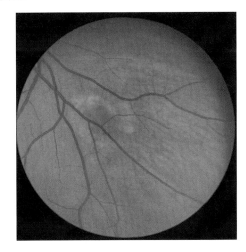

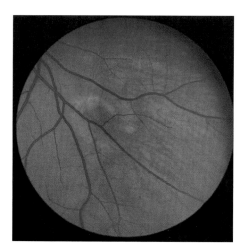

◄ 163
This lesion had been present for a number of years and was totally asymptomatic. What is the most likely diagnosis?

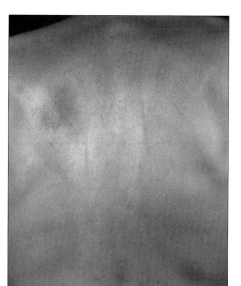

◄ 164
These plaque-like lesions had been present over a number of months. There were no associated systemic symptoms or signs. Suggest a likely diagnosis.

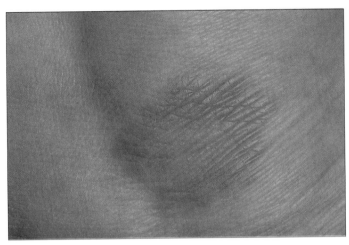

▲ 165
This lesion had an insidious onset. The patient has diabetes mellitus. What diagnosis is suggested?

166 ▶
(a) What is the diagnosis?
(b) List two associations.

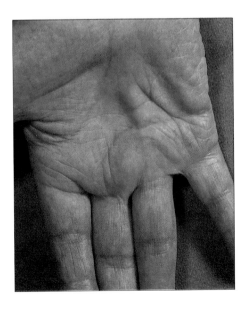

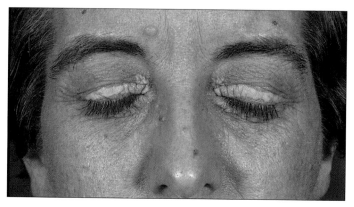

▲ 167
(a) What physical signs are present on this patient's face?
(b) Suggest a unifying underlying diagnosis.

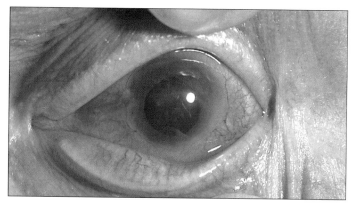

▲ 168
This is the eye of a 68-year-old man presenting with a two-week history of soreness of both eyes and pains in the hands and lower legs. His erythrocyte sedimentation rate was 105 mm/h and his Venereal Disease Research Laboratory (VDRL) test was positive with a negative treponemal haemagglutination (TPHA) test.
(a) What physical signs are present?
(b) What is the differential diagnosis?

169 ▶

These are the legs of a patient
with joint pains associated with
microscopic haematuria. What
is the most likely diagnosis?

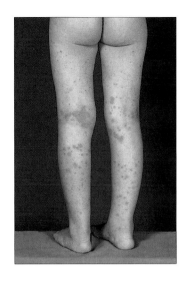

170 ▶

These are the legs of a young
adult presenting with recurrent
epistaxis and widespread non-
branching purpuric lesions on
the arms and legs. She was
otherwise in good health, but
had a previous history of
thyrotoxicosis. What is the
most likely diagnosis?

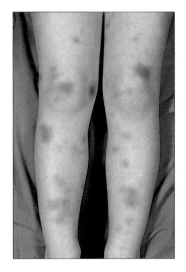

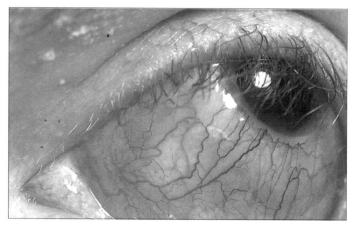

▲ 171

This is the eye of a patient under investigation for weight loss, fever, and coughing. A pulmonary lesion was present. What is the most likely diagnosis?

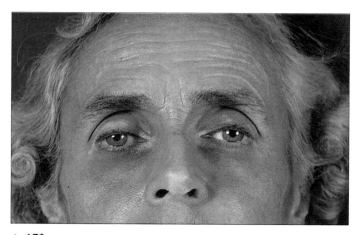

▲ 172

This is the face of a patient who complained of intense pruritus and whose biochemical investigations revealed a persistently raised alkaline phosphatase. What is the most likely diagnosis?

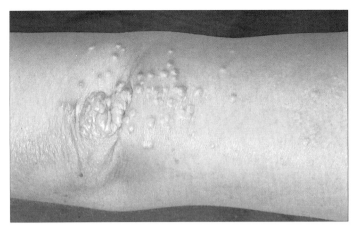

▲ 173
What lesions are shown?

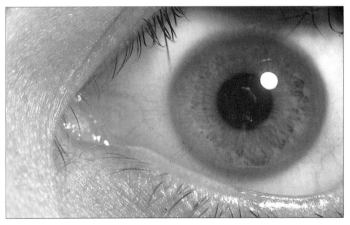

▲ 174
What diagnosis is suggested by the ocular appearance of this patient who presented with a severe haemolytic crisis and who had abnormal liver function tests?

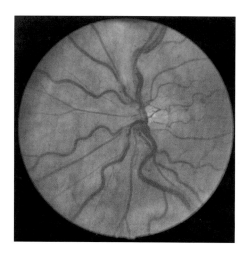

◀ 175
What is the
diagnosis?

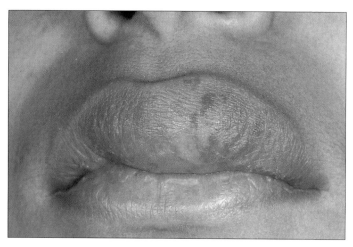

▲ 176
This abnormality had been present since birth. What is the
diagnosis?

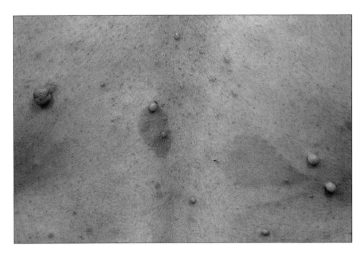

▲ 177
(a) What is the diagnosis?
(b) List two associations.

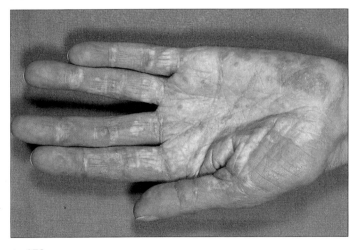

▲ 178
(a) What lesions are shown?
(b) List one association.

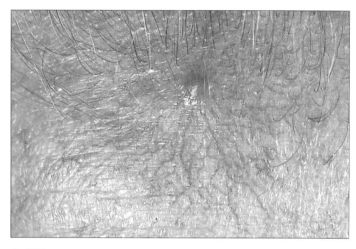

▲ 179
(a) What lesion is demonstrated?
(b) List two associations.

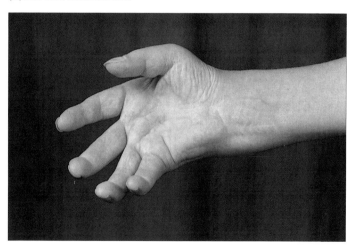

▲ 180
What is the most likely cause of this appearance?

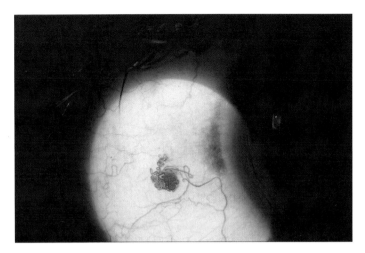

▲ 181
List two abnormalities on this conjunctiva.

182 ▶
(a) What is the diagnosis?
(b) List two associations.

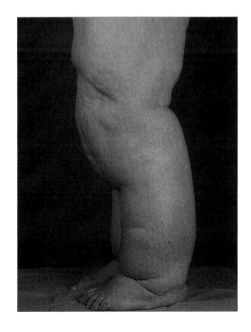

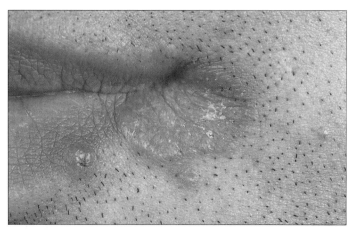

▲ 183
This patient was suffering from a chronic respiratory complaint with a reduced KLCO (corrected diffusion capacity for carbon monoxide) and had hypercalcaemia and hypercalciuria. What is the most likely cause of the chronic lesion at the angle of the mouth?

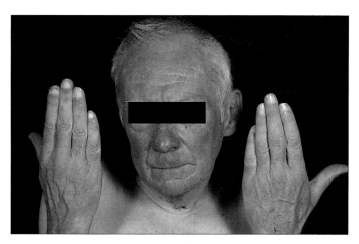

▲ 184
This man complained of itching skin following hot baths. What is the most likely diagnosis?

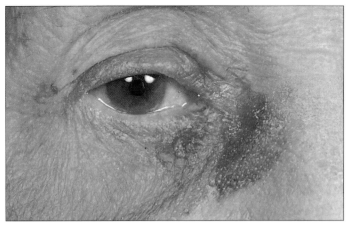

▲ 185

This is the appearance of a man with heavy proteinuria, and dislipidaemia. What underlying diagnosis is suggested by this appearance?

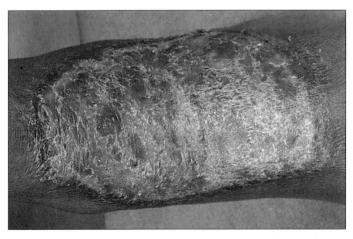

▲ 186

What is the most likely infective agent causing these appearances?

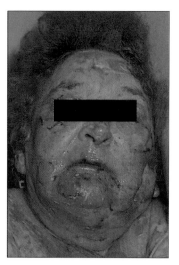

◀ 187
This patient developed an acute cutaneous illness following antibiotic treatment. What is the likely diagnosis?

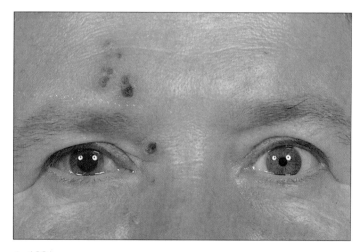

▲ 188
(a) What is the diagnosis?
(b) What is the treatment?

189 ▶

(a) What lesions are shown?

(b) What is an important
association?

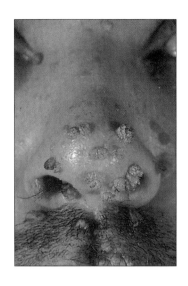

190 ▶

This is the appearance of a
neonate's foot. What diagnosis
is suggested by this appearance?

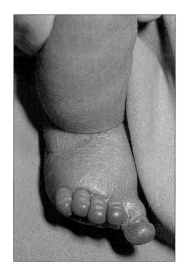

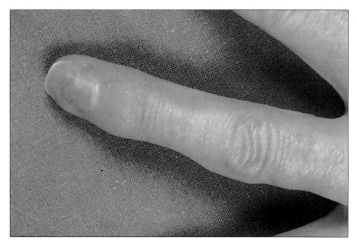

▲ 191
What dermatological condition is suggested by this appearance?

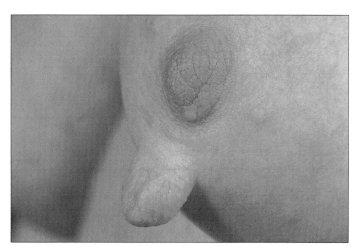

▲ 192
What is the most likely cause of this unusual appearance?

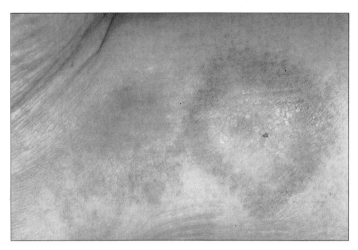

▲ 193
This eruption was of fairly sudden onset. What is the most likely
diagnosis?

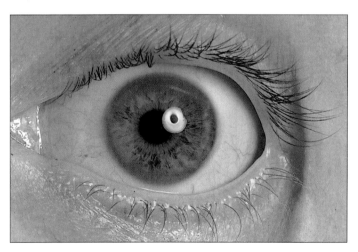

▲ 194
What is the diagnosis?

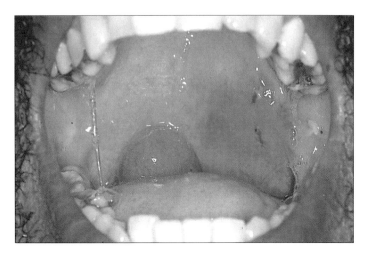

▲ 195
What is the diagnosis?

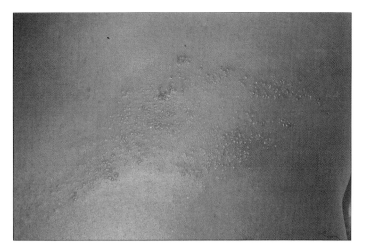

▲ 196
What is the diagnosis?

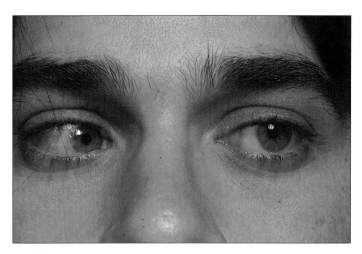

▲ 197

This patient was attempting to gaze to the left. What lesion is shown?

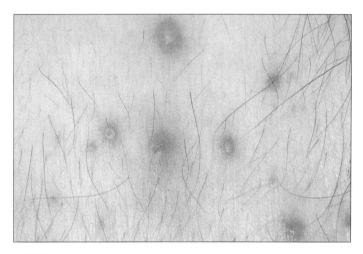

▲ 198

This was part of a more generalized eruption presenting in a 25-year-old man who had a constitutional illness with a fever. What is the most likely diagnosis?

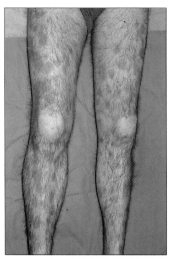

◀ 199
This cutaneous appearance occurred in a man with known immunodeficiency and a susceptibility to infection. What is the likely diagnosis?

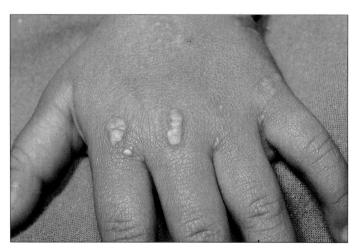

▲ 200
(a) What lesions are shown?
(b) What investigations are required?

1 (a) Erythema nodosum.
   (b) This may occur following sulphonamide therapy or streptococcal infection, and in association with early tuberculosis.

2 Pellagra. This case may have been secondary to isoniazid therapy.

3 Systemic sclerosis. Telangiectatic lesions can be seen on the face, as well as pinching of the nose and fine skin folds around the mouth.

4 Dry macular degeneration.

5 Lupus pernio. This is one of the cutaneous manifestations of sarcoidosis.

6 Target cells are plentiful. This can occur in a number of conditions, in this case, following splenectomy.

7 (a) Angioid streaks. These are large breaks in Bruch's membrane.
   (b) They are associated with Paget's disease, acromegaly, pseudoxanthoma elasticum, sickle cell disease, and severe myopia.

8 Gonadal dysgenesis (Turner's syndrome—XO chromosomes).

9 Relapsing polychondritis, syphilis, and Wegener's granulomatosis, may cause this physical sign.

10 These are the appearances of a child with rickets. The lower limbs show considerable bowing.

11 (a) High arch palate.
   (b) This may be associated with Marfan's syndrome.

12 Testicular feminization (androgen insensitivity syndrome) or Leydig cell hypoplasia is an alternative diagnosis.

13 Recurrent thyroglossal cyst.

14 Eruptive xanthomata. These may occur in familial lipoprotein lipase deficiency, causing an elevation of chylomicrons. It may be associated with pancreatitis.

15 This shows an intra-abdominal testis, which is not infrequently found in testicular feminization.

16 Splenic and portal vein thrombosis, with a demonstrable portosystemic shunt.

17 This is probably a cutaneous vasculitis. Henoch–Schönlein purpura should be excluded, although in many cases this may be an isolated cutaneous vasculitis. Dapsone has been tried in a number of patients with these isolated cutaneous lesions with rare anecdotal reports of success.

18 (a) Koilonychia. This is a spooning of the nails.
(b) It is associated with iron deficiency anaemia. Other features of iron deficiency include glossitis with a reddened, swollen, smooth, shiny tongue, angular stomatitis, gastric atrophy with achlorhydria and, occasionally, a postcricoid web (Plummer–Vinson syndrome).

19 Osler–Weber–Rendu disease (hereditary haemorrhagic telangiectasia). This is an inherited autosomal dominant disorder in which there are frequent episodes of nasal and gastrointestinal bleeding from abnormal telangiectatic capillaries.

20 (a) Eruptive xanthomata. These may be seen in familial lipoprotein lipase deficiency (with elevation of chylomicrons) and rarely in familial hypertriglyceridaemia due to the low-density lipoprotein excess.
(b) The patient should have a complete lipoprotein electrophoretic screen.

21 (a) These are striae.
(b) They may be seen in association with Cushing's syndrome, but more commonly, simple obesity in a pale-skinned individual.

22 (a) Glossitis with mild angular stomatitis is demonstrated.
(b) The patient should be investigated for possible underlying iron deficiency anaemia.

23 Transfusion haemosiderosis with increased pigmentation of the hand. The ferritin level in this case exceeded 3000 mg/l.

24 Hereditary methaemoglobinaemia. This may be due either to the presence of one of the methaemoglobins or a deficiency of the enzyme cytochrome B5-reductase. In contrast to the induction of methaemoglobinaemia by drugs or toxins, which can be life-threatening, this patient had few symptoms. If methaemoglobin exceeds 15 g/l (10% of the total haemoglobin), affected individuals have clinically obvious cyanosis. The colour of the skin is indistinguishable from the much more common cyanosis due to impaired oxygen saturation, which occurs in pulmonary and cardiac disorders.

25 Beta-thalassaemia major. This shows the characteristic facies of a boy, including prominent maxillae, widening of the bridge of the nose, and often marked bossing of the frontal and parietal bones.

26 Graft versus host disease (GVHD). Some degree of GVHD occurs in all patients receiving bone marrow transplantation. In about 10%, however, a chronic phase may ensue, with the onset of a dry cough, mucositis, dyspnoea, and airflow obstruction in the small airways. Chest radiographs may reveal peribronchial infiltrates. Maculopapular eruptions are common in acute GVHD. In this condition, lesions frequently begin on the palms and soles. In contrast, lichen planus-like lesions are also observed in chronic GVHD.

27 (a) This shows tufting of the terminal phalanx and subperiosteal erosions.
(b) The appearances are most in keeping with primary hyperparathyroidism, and hypercalcaemia is likely.

28 (a) Gum hyperplasia.
(b) This may occur with myeloblastic leukaemia, phenytoin usage, cyclosporin usage, and thalassaemias.

29 (a) *Candida* infection in the mouth is not infrequent in such immunosuppressed patients.
(b) Treatment may be either nystatin lozenges or amphotericin lozenges.

30 Paget's disease. There is curvature and bowing of the femur and, not atypically, the disease is patchy in its distribution.

31 This is a cutaneous manifestation of graft versus host disease.

32 Acute haemarthrosis. This case was caused by recurrent bleeding within the knee of a haemophiliac.

33 Volkmann's ischaemic contracture.

34 Synovial cyst.

35 A phaeochromocytoma. Incision of the lesion will generally show haemorrhagic necrotic areas.

36 Dermatitis herpetiformis. This an intensively pruritic, chronic, papulovesicular skin rash caused by lesions that are symmetrically distributed over the extensor surfaces (elbows, knees, buttocks, back, scalp, and posterior neck). Because pruritus is prominent, patients may present with excoriations and crusted papules, but no observable primary lesions. Almost all patients have an associated, usually subclinical, gluten-sensitive enteropathy and more than 90% express the HLA B8 DRW3 and HLA DQW2 haplotypes. The disease is typically chronic.

37 A pseudoarthritis of the left humerus. This resulted from non-union of a fracture.

38 (a) There is considerable synovial thickening, ulnar deviation, some swan-neck deformity, wasting of the small muscles of the hands, and swelling of the wrist joints.
(b) The diagnosis is rheumatoid arthritis.

39 (a) Clawing of the toes.
(b) This may be seen in chronic peripheral neuritis, Charcot–Marie–Tooth syndrome, and Friedreich's ataxia.

40 Massively increased uptake of radionuclide. This is most in keeping with metabolic bone disease.

41 (a) Vitiligo.
(b) This is a non-organ-specific marker of autoimmune disease. It may be associated with Graves' disease, Addison's disease, and primary biliary cirrhosis.

42 (a) Adenoma sebaceum (tuberous sclerosis).
(b) This may be associated with epilepsy.

43 (a) This is scleromalacia.

(b) It is usually seen in the context of episcleritis and is commonly associated with rheumatoid arthritis and other connective tissue diseases.

44 (a) Arthritis mutilans.

(b) This is associated with severe psoriasis.

45 Cutaneous sarcoid.

46 Seborrhoeic wart. This is quite benign and does not require excision.

47 Pityriasis lichenoid chronicum.

48 (a) Ligamentous laxity.

(b) This may be associated with osteogenesis imperfecta, Marfan's syndrome, or Ehlers–Danlos syndrome.

49 (a) Polydactyly.

(b) There is an association with congenital heart disease.

50 (a) Joint laxity.

(b) In this context, it is probably related to osteogenesis imperfecta.

51 Haemochromatosis. The slate-grey pigmentation is associated with melanin deposition in the skin. Other features of haemochromatosis include hypogonadism and disturbances of the hypothalamo–pituitary axis, as well as cardiomyopathy.

52 This is a simple cyst of the foreskin, which is entirely benign.

53 (a) Leukoplakia.

(b) This may be premalignant.

54 A giant hairy naevus.

55 Onychogryphosis.

56 A strawberry naevus.

57 Sister Joseph's nodule.

58 Central retinal artery occlusion. The areas supplied by the cilioretinal arteries have preserved the normal vascular pattern of part of the retina nearest to the optic disc.

59 Discoid eczema.

60 (a) Onychomycosis.
(b) The patient could be treated with a prolonged course of griseofulvin.

61 Fanconi's anaemia. Patients with Fanconi's anaemia usually have a normal or nearly normal blood count at birth and during infancy. The disease presents with the effects of pancytopenia, usually at about five years of age or later. Bleeding due to thrombocytopenia is the commonest presentation, with anaemia second. The bone marrow becomes progressively hypocellular over the years. Dyserythropoiesis is common. Associated abnormalities include hypopigmentation of the skin and malformations of the skeleton (aplasia or hypoplasia of the thumb and aplasia or hypoplasia of the radii). Cryptorchism is present in 20% of cases.

62 Molluscum contagiosum. These lesions were present in a patient with acquired immunodeficiency syndrome (AIDS). Molluscum contagiosum is caused by an unclassified pox virus that cannot be cultured *in vitro*. Lesions occur anywhere on the body except on the palms and soles, and appear as pearly, flesh-coloured, raised, umbilicated nodules. They generally appear in crops, are painless, and resolve over a period of weeks to several years. Spread is probably by direct contact, which accounts for the commonly observed genital distribution of lesions in sexually active adults. No specific therapy is available, although lesions can be removed by curettage.

63 This is a typical appearance of dermatomyositis. The most common manifestation of this condition is a purple–red discoloration of the upper eyelids, sometimes associated with scaling (heliotrope erythema) and periorbital oedema. Erythema and scaling may be particularly prominent over the elbows, knees, and the dorsal interphalangeal joints, as shown here. Approximately one-third of patients have violaceous flat-topped papules over the dorsal interphalangeal joints, which are pathognomonic of dermatomyositis (Gottron's sign or Gottron's papules). These lesions can be contrasted with the erythema and scaling of the dorsum of the fingers in some patients with systemic lupus erythematosus, which spares the skin over the interphalangeal joints. Periungual telangiectasia may be prominent, and a lacy or reticulated erythema may be associated with fine scaling on the extensor surfaces of the thighs and upper arms.

64 These grey–white, non-pruritic, scaly lesions are the typical lesions of psoriasis.

65 Henoch–Schönlein purpura. This is the most common of the hypersensitivity vasculitides, and is characterized by a palpable purpura, most commonly distributed over the buttocks and lower extremities. In addition, arthralgia, gastrointestinal signs and symptoms, and glomerulonephritis may occur. The disease is usually seen in children and has a remarkable tendency to resolve and recur several times over a period of weeks or months, usually ending in spontaneous resolution. A number of antigens have been implicated in the immunopathogenesis of the disease, including infectious agents, drugs, certain foods, insect bites, and immunizations. Immunoglobulin A is the antibody class most often seen in the immune complexes of these patients.

66 These are the purplish-violaceous lesions of Kaposi's sarcoma. Where the disease is limited either no treatment or a local course of irradiation may be appropriate.

67 Budd–Chiari syndrome. The prominent abdominal wall veins may be due to portal hypertension or to collaterals passing an inferior vena caval block. The condition is usually due to hepatic vein occlusion, and ultrasound and computerized tomography may suggest hepatic venous occlusion and distension of the portal circulation with portal collaterals. The usual pattern on a technetium radioisotope liver scan is diffuse patchy uptake with, more unusually, an enhanced uptake, which is essentially due to candate lobe enlargement. Budd–Chiari syndrome is associated with haematological disorders, malignancy, oral contraception in women, and antitumour therapy, and rarely occurs in pregnancy and in the first part of the period.

68 Impetigo. This appears to be the result of direct or indirect inoculation of the organism.

69 (a) Vitreous haemorrhage.
   (b) Diabetic retinopathy (neovascularization).

70 Perniosis. This is a vasculitic disorder associated with cold exposure. Various erythematous lesions develop in association with pruritus and a burning sensation. Occasionally, blistering and ulceration may occur. Pathological examination demonstrates angiitis, which is characterized by intimal proliferation and perivascular infiltration of mononuclear and polymorphonuclear leucocytes. Giant cells may be present in the subcutaneous tissue. Patients should avoid exposure to cold.

71 (a) Extensive port wine stains.
(b) No medical therapy will improve this appearance, but laser treatment may help.

72 Beau's lines.

73 Cutis verticis gyrata.

74 Purpura. This case was associated with severe thrombocytopenia.

75 Melasma. This is usually a symmetrical brown patch on the face, especially the cheeks, upper lip, and forehead. Similar changes are seen in pregnancy and in the adult form of Gaucher's disease. In the last group there is also hyperpigmentation of the distal lower extremities.

76 Multiple scrotal cysts. These are entirely benign.

77 Psoriatic arthropathy. Both the articular manifestations (arthritis mutilans, distal arthropathy) are shown, together with clear evidence of psoriatic nail disease.

78 Xanthelasma, bilateral ptosis.

79 Basal cell carcinoma. The rolled edges with telangiectatic lesions on the surface are typical.

80 (a) Bilateral exophthalmos is noted.
(b) This is a feature of dysthyroid eye disease and may be associated with underlying thyrotoxicosis.

81 Squamous cell carcinoma.

82 Pemphigus vulgaris. This disorder is characterized by the loss of cohesion between epidermal cells, a process known as acantholysis, with the resultant formation of intraepidermal blisters. Clinical lesions of pemphigus vulgaris typically consist of flaccid blisters on either normal-appearing or erythematous skin. Manual pressure to the skin of these patients will illustrate the separation of the epidermis (so-called Nikolsky's sign). In more than 50% of patients, the lesions begin in the mouth, and over 90% of patients have oromucocutaneous involvement at some time during their disease.

83 Cutaneous horn.

84 Molluscum contagiosum.

85 Thyroglossal cyst.

86 Multiple seborrhoeic keratoses.

87 Toxic epidermal necrolysis. This is a serious cutaneous drug reaction, and may be fatal. Drugs are most frequently the cause, and the onset is generally acute and characterized by epidermal necrosis with a minimal dermal inflammatory process. Drugs implicated include sulphonamides, anticonvulsants, non-steroidal anti-inflammatory agents and allopurinol, and more rarely phenytoin and measles vaccine.

88 Sarcoidosis. The classical cutaneous nodules are demonstrated here.

89 Psoriasis of the nail. This shows a typical appearance of onycholysis with thimble pitting.

90 Systemic lupus erythematosus. These hands show photosensitive eruptions, particularly over the knuckles.

91 An arteriovenous fistula. This may have been created for dialysis.

92 Haemangioma of the lip.

93 Hutchinson's freckle.

94 Diffuse systemic sclerosis. The appearance is that of sclerodactyly, with contractures of the hands.

95 Erythema nodosum. This can occur with tuberculosis, sarcoidosis, leprosy, and a large range of microbial agents. Drugs commonly associated with erythema nodosum include sulphonamides; the oral contraceptive pill may also be responsible.

96 (a) These are Kayser–Fleischer rings.
(b) They represent copper deposition within Descemet's membrane and are associated with Wilson's disease.

97 Pyoderma gangrenosum. There is a clear-cut association with inflammatory bowel disease.

98 Morphoea. This is a form of scleroderma in which there are well-demarcated lesions within the skin, a separate disease to disseminated sclerosis. Some patients may have extensive confluent areas of skin involvement, giving rise to generalized morphoea.

99 Herpes zoster infection (shingles).

100 Lichen planus. This is a papulosquamous disorder in which the primary lesions are pruritic, polygonal, flat-topped, and violaceous and are covered with a network of greyish lines (Wickham's striae). The lesions have a predilection for the wrists, shins, lower back, and genitalia. Lichen planus can occur on the buccal mucosa, where it can present as a net-like whitish eruption. Histological examination of the lesions demonstrates hyperkeratosis, irregular acanthosis, a band-like dermal infiltrate of the lymphocytes adjacent to the epidermis, and damage to the epidermal basal cells. Most patients have a spontaneous remission six months to two years after the onset of the disease and topical glucocorticoids are the mainstay of therapy.

101 This case was caused by *Aspergillus niger*, a mould with septate hyphae about 2–4 mm in diameter. The fungus is identified by its growth and microscopic appearance in culture. Tetracycline can cause a similar blackening of the tongue.

102 Bowen's disease. This represents a squamous cell carcinoma *in situ* and usually presents as a single lesion. The plaque is well demarcated, pink to red in colour, and the amount of scale varies. It is found in both exposed and protected areas of the body. The possibility of arsenic exposure should be explored in these patients and the palms and soles should be examined for arsenic keratosis.

103 Basal cell carcinoma. The rolled edges with an ulcerated central pit are characteristic. Cryosurgery or 5-fluorouracil cream may be used here or, most effectively, a short course of superficial X-ray therapy.

104 Vasculitic rash. This might occur in the context of a connective tissue disease.

105 Pemphigoid. This is a subepidermal blistering disease and is usually seen in the elderly. Lesions typically consist of tense blisters on either normal-appearing or erythematous skin. Pruritus may be non-existent or severe. As lesions evolve, tense blisters tend to rupture and be replaced by flaccid lesions or erosions with or without surmounting crusts. Non-traumatized blisters heal without scarring. Biopsies of inflammatory lesions typically show an eosinophilic leucocytic infiltrate within the papillary dermis at the site of vesicle formation and in perivascular areas.

106 Ophthalmic Graves' disease. In addition this patient has a conjunctival inflammatory lesion on the right.

107 Actinic melanosis. The pigmented lesions are present on sun-exposed areas and are a consequence of chronic sun exposure.

108 Pterygium.

109 Thyroglossal cyst. This lesion moves on swallowing and is a cystic lesion derived from the embryonic thyroglossal duct. It is entirely benign.

110 (a) Congenital adrenal hyperplasia.
(b) 17-alpha-hydroxyprogesterone should be measured and a urinary steroid profile obtained.

111 Melanosis oculi. This is an entirely benign lesion.

112 Medullated nerve fibres. These are entirely benign.

113 Episcleritis with evidence of scleromalacia in the left eye (bluish discoloration of the sclera).

114 (a) Bluish pigmentation of the cartilage.
(b) The diagnosis here is ochronosis.

115 Monoliasis of the penis (monoliasis balanitis). Urine sugar should be tested in all such cases.

116 Erythema induratum (Bazin's disease). The condition predominates in females aged between 10 and 20 years. Pathologically, there is a nonspecific or tuberculoid infiltrate in the lower part of the dermis. Proliferative changes occur and caseation, which accounts for the clinical breakdown of the lesions, may follow. The lesions are notably painless and, when they break down, ulcerate and leave scars. The edges of the ulcers are steep or undermined. Lesions may persist for months.

117 Sycosis barbae. A persistent folliculitis of the beard area, sycosis barbae is primarily a foreign body reaction to hair with secondary infection, which is sometimes caused by *Staphylococcus aureus*, but more often *S. epidermidis*. If the subcutaneous tissue becomes involved in a staphyloccal infection, a boil or furuncle results.

118 Primary herpes simplex lesion of the face.

119 There is exophthalmos of the right eye, most likely due to dysthyroid eye disease. This not uncommonly affects only one eye.

120 Pyogenic granuloma.

121 (a) Onycholysis.
(b) In this case, it was due to thyrotoxicosis, but it may also occur in onychomycosis and psoriasis.

122 (a) Granuloma annulare. This is a partial necrosis of the collagen and keratin cells associated with immunoglobulin and complement deposition, resulting in a lymphocytic and histiocytic response known as palisading granuloma. This is entirely reversible over many months and years in granuloma annulare and is associated with insulin-dependent diabetes mellitus. Widespread forms of granuloma annulare are often of the giant-type, forming large violaceous plaques or rings.
(b) No treatment is necessary as eventual resolution is expected in 75% of cases within two years, but intralesional corticosteroids probably speed resolution.

123 Old choroiditis. This may occur in sarcoidosis, old toxoplasmosis, and old *Toxocara* infection.

124 Osler–Weber–Rendu disease (hereditary haemorrhagic telangiectasia).

125 (a) Hard exudates are shown, with occasional dot haemorrhages.
(b) The patient had underlying diabetes mellitus.

126 Alopecia areata. The onset of this condition is nearly always sudden, and often there is a hair loss occurring overnight. Regrowth of hair is usual, but not a certainty.

127 Discoid lupus erythematosus. These are often violaceous, hyper-pigmented, atrophic plaques, often with evidence of follicular plugging, which generally results in scarring. Alopecia is a not infrequent finding.

128 Acute iritis and scleritis.

129 Dermatitis herpetiformis. This is an intensely pruritic, chronic papulovesicular skin disease characterized by lesions that are symmetrically distributed over the extensor surfaces. The primary lesion is a papule or urticarial plaque, which is frequently excoriated as a result of intense pruritus. Almost all patients have an associated, usually subclinical, gluten-sensitive enteropathy, and more than 90% express the HLA DRW3 and HLA DQW2 haplotypes. The disease is usually chronic.

130 Molluscum contagiosum.

131 Simple conjunctival cysts. These give the appearance of chemosis.

132 Ringworm infection (tinea corporis). The lesion is typically annular in type, producing red ring lesions, with tiny peripheral vesicles and a clear slightly scaly centre. The diagnosis is made by microscopy. Canesten cream (clotrimazole 1%) may be used for treatment.

133 This is tinea capitis. The treatment is as detailed in **132**.

134 Malignant melanoma. There is a rolled edge, and an irregular outline with variable pigmentation within the lesion. This appearance is virtually diagnostic.

135 Bowen's disease.

136 Pemphigoid.

137 (a) This is a gouty tophus.
(b) It is associated with significant hyperuricaemia. Chronic tophaceous gouty arthritis inevitably follows recurrent acute attacks and is characterized by asymmetrical joint swelling. Tophi are typically found in the articular tissues, the cartilaginous helix of the ear, bursae, and tendon sheaths. Tophus formation is related to the serum urate concentration and local factors, but is not seen in individuals with asymptomatic hyperuricaemia.

138 (a) Atrophic glossitis.
(b) This may be found in severe iron deficiency anaemia or in vitamin B_{12} deficiency.

139 Keratoacanthoma of the eyelid.

140 Necrotic vasculitis. This patient had polyarteritis nodosa.

141 These are the lesions of macular retinochoroiditis. These could be caused by toxoplasmosis or sarcoidosis.

142 (a) Papilloedema in a chronic setting.
(b) This may be associated with a constriction of peripheral vision.

143 Orbital amyloidosis. Amyloid deposits in the capillary beds will cause fragility of the vessels. When purpuric lesions occur around the eyes, the expression periorbital palpable purpura (raccoon facies) is sometimes used.

144 Lichen planus.

145 This is an episcleritic lesion associated with rheumatoid arthritis. Episcleritis is one of the ocular manifestations of rheumatoid arthritis. Severe lesions may lead to thinning of the sclera, resulting eventually in scleromalacia perforans.

146 (a) Multiple viral warts.
(b) These may be treated by curettage or intralesional interferon therapy.

147 (a) Pinguecula.
(b) This is asymptomatic and no treatment is necessary unless it interferes with vision.

148 Cutaneous leishmaniasis. This patient had been bitten by sandfly. The initial lesion is an erythematous nodule developing at the site of the bite, followed by a thin golden crust. The nodule reaches its final size, usually 1–5 cm in diameter, over weeks or months. The crust may remain superficial or thicken to replace the nodule, or may fall away leaving an ulcer with a raised edge. Satellite papules are common. After months, or years, the lesions start to heal, leaving a depressed mottled scar. Lesions can often be healed using a thermostatically controlled pad or water sack generating temperatures of 40–42°C.

149 (a) Cutaneous calcification.
(b) This may be associated with dermatomyositis and systemic sclerosis.

150 Anisocoria. Asymmetrical pupil diameters are not common.

151 (a) Mild diversion squint, exophthalmos, left tarsorrhaphy.
(b) The patient has ophthalmic Graves' disease.

152 Hypertensive retinopathy with haemorrhages. There is considerable sclerosis of the arterioles with some superficial haemorrhages; a more recent haemorrhage can be seen around the macula.

153 Old healed choroiditis. Old toxoplasmosis or *Toxocara* infection may account for this appearance.

154 Kaposi's sarcoma. A variety of neoplastic and premalignant diseases occur with an increased frequency in human immunodeficiency virus (HIV)-infected individuals. Kaposi's sarcoma is a multicentric neoplasm consisting of multiple vascular nodules and occurs in the skin, mucous membranes, and viscera. The course ranges from indolent, with only minor skin or lymph node involvement, to fulminant, with extensive cutaneous and visceral involvement. Kaposi's sarcoma is an early manifestation of HIV infection, at times occurring in patients of normal CD4-positive cell counts. From the pathological perspective, Kaposi's sarcoma is probably more a consequence of disordered cytokine regulation of cell growth. Usually the tumour respects tissue planes and is rarely invasive.

155 (a) Bilateral dense arcus senilis.
(b) This may be associated with dislipidaemia, particularly familial combined dislipidaemia.

156 Active episcleritis.

157 (a) Splinter haemorrhages.
(b) These were present in a patient with subacute bacterial endocarditis. They probably represent vasculitic lesions in the nail bed.

158 (a) Neurofibromatosis.
(b) This patient had a phaeochromocytoma removed from the right adrenal. Phaeochromocytomas occur in 1% of patients with neurofibromatosis.

159 Condyloma acuminata (venereal warts). These can be treated with podophyllin, but it is also important to treat the patient's partner.

160 This is most likely to be a tuberculous node.

161 (a) Acanthosis nigricans.

(b) This may occur in acromegaly, severe insulin resistance states, and the Prader–Willi syndrome.

162 Cystinosis. This is sometimes associated with photophobia due to refractile corneal opacities. Cystine crystals also accumulate under the conjunctiva. In this condition, the peripheral part of the retina may show pigmentary degeneration, most marked in the temporal quadrants. The diagnosis of cystinosis is usually confirmed by demonstrating cystine crystals in a bone marrow aspirate, in leucocytes, or by a conjunctival biopsy. In this condition, real tubular damage produces a Fanconi syndrome, acidosis, and tubular proteinuria, with an excess of gammaglobulin light chains.

163 Simple retinal naevus.

164 Macular amyloid. This is one of three forms of amyloidosis, but it is limited to the skin. The other two are lichenoid amyloidosis (usually affecting the lower extremities) and nodular amyloidosis. In macular and lichenoid amyloidosis, the deposits are composed of altered epidermal keratin. Recently, macular amyloidosis has been associated with multiple endocrine neoplasia type 2A.

165 Granuloma annulare.

166 (a) Dupuytren's contractures.

(b) These may be a feature of chronic alcoholic liver disease, but may be idiopathic.

167 (a) The patient has xanthelasma, is jaundiced, and has a number of spider naevi.

(b) The most likely diagnosis is primary biliary cirrhosis.

168 (a) There is an active uveitis, associated with loss of the eyelashes.

(b) The combination of polyarthritis and uveitis suggests a seronegative arthritis. These include Reiter's syndrome, systemic lupus erythematosus, sarcoidosis, or an immune complex disease. In this case, the patient had lepromatous leprosy.

169 Henoch–Schönlein (anaphylactoid) purpura.

170 Idiopathic thrombocytopenic purpura (ITP). The onset is usually explosive and follows recovery from a viral illness. In most cases (60%), recovery occurs within 4–6 weeks, and 90% of patients will recover within 3–6 months. Transient immunological thrombocytopenia can also complicate some cases of infectious mononucleosis, acute toxoplasmosis, or cytomegalovirus infection and can be part of the prodromal phase of viral hepatitis. There is an association between thrombocytopenic purpura and thyrotoxicosis.

171 Tuberculous uveitis. Tuberculosis is associated with a granulomatous chronic iridocyclitis, and occasionally a retinal vasculitis. Any patient with a chronic iridocyclitis should have a Mantoux test and evidence of tuberculosis should be sought.

172 Primary biliary cirrhosis. The pigmented skin is typical and the elevated alkaline phosphatase may precede an elevation of serum bilirubin by many years.

173 These are eruptive xanthomata on the elbows. They are seen in type I or type IV dislipidaemias.

174 Wilson's disease. Kayser–Fleischer corneal rings are demonstrated. This is a granular deposit of copper, probably as copper proteinate, in the deep layers of Descemet's membrane. The usual colour is brown, but rarely a heavy pigment deposit seen over a brown iris may appear grey. The pigment is always densest at the top crescent of the cornea from 10 o'clock to 2 o'clock. It then appears in the lower crescent, and these two crescents extend laterally to join and form complete rings, which are therefore a rather late manifestation of the disease. Corneal pigment is invariably present in the neurological stage, and may be seen in the hepatic or even in the presymptomatic stages of the illness. Another less common ocular manifestation of Wilson's disease is the sunflower cataract due to copper deposits in the lens.

175 Papilloedema. The disc margins are indistinct, and the veins are dilated, tortuous, and congested.

176 Haemangioma of the lip.

177 (a) Neurofibromatosis.
    (b) Associated conditions include phaeochromocytoma, sarcomatous degeneration, and acoustic neuroma.

178 (a) Planar xanthomata.
(b) They may be associated with primary biliary cirrhosis.

179 (a) Spider angioma.
(b) This may be associated with chronic liver disease or use of the contraceptive pill.

180 Chronic rheumatoid arthritis involving the hand. There shows substantial ulnar deviation, small muscle wasting of the hands, some palmar erythema, and the classical deformities of the rheumatoid hand.

181 Right conjunctival haemangioma and melanosis oculi. Neither lesion requires any specific therapy and the patient should be reassured.

182 (a) Bilateral lymphoedema of the legs.
(b) This may occur in Milroy's disease as well as in the tropics as elephantiasis due to filariasis.

183 Cutaneous sarcoid. Sarcoidosis would link all the abnormalities demonstrated by this patient.

184 Polycythaemia rubra vera. The plethoric facies and red coloration of the hands are typical. Polycythaemia can occur as part of a primary myeloproliferative disorder or can be secondary to a number of lesions including chronic respiratory disease, stress polycythaemia, cerebral haemangioma, the Pickwickian syndrome, abnormal haemoglobins, and abnormal 2-3 diphosphoglycerate metabolism.

185 Amyloidosis. Capillary fragility, particularly around the eyes, leads to purpura with minimal trauma.

186 A fungal infection.

187 Toxic epidermal necrolysis. This is the most serious cutaneous drug reaction possible, and may be fatal. The onset is generally acute and is characterized by epidermal necrosis with a minimal dermal inflammatory process. This reaction is often associated with sulphonamides, anticonvulsants, non-steroidal anti-inflammatory drugs, and allopurinol.

188 (a) Herpes ophthalmicus.
(b) The patient could be treated with high-dose acyclovir early in the course of the disease.

189 (a) Cutaneous warts.
(b) These are either iatrogenic or, more likely, a feature of acquired immunodeficiency syndrome (AIDS).

190 Lymphoedema is present, and this is suggestive of Turner's syndrome.

191 Psoriasis. Both the nail and the distal interphalangeal joints are affected.

192 Neurofibromatosis.

193 Erythema multiforme. Some target lesions are shown.

194 Kayser–Fleischer rings in Wilson's disease.

195 Uvulitis. Inflammation of the soft palate and uvula sometimes occurs in association with smoking marijuana.

196 Herpes zoster infection (shingles).

197 Left sixth nerve palsy.

198 Chickenpox.

199 Job's–Luke syndrome.

200 (a) Xanthomata (eruptive) over the dorsum of the hands.
(b) Lipid levels should be checked.

INDEX

Numbers refer to Question and Answer numbers.